Sugar Free Recipes

52 Low Carb Low Sugar Recipes

© 2015 by Peggy Annear
Published by Kangaroo Flat Books

Visit the Author's Page

for the full color, linked Kindle/PC book format.

http://www.amazon.com/author/peggy-annear

ISBN-13: 978-0-9925435-5-6

ISBN-10: 099254355X

Introduction.. 7

    How to Remove Sugar from Your Diet! 8

    What about Honey?.. 12

    How to Understand Sugar Amounts on Labels.............. 12

    Check the Total Carbohydrates...................................... 13

    What is an Acceptable Amount of Carbs? 14

The Google Search Method 16

The Low Sugar Myth 17

Low Sugar Fruits.. 19

High Sugar Fruits... 20

Vegetables High in Sugars.. 21

Vegetables Low in Sugar 22

Low Sugar Milks.. 25

The Problem with Fructose 27

High Fructose Foods 29

    Low Fructose Fruits and Vegetables............................. 30

    Moderate Fructose Fruits & Vegetables........................ 31

    High Fructose Fruits... 32

    Variety is Key... 34

The French Connection.. 35

    Nut & Seed Granola 36

    Apricot Smoothie 38

    Savory French Toast.. 39

    Apple Pie Oatmeal 40

    Almond Flour Crepes... 41

http://www.amazon.com/author/peggy-annear

Kale Smoothie Blend 42

Eggnog 43

Vegetable V8 Drink 44

Lunch Smoothie 44

Oven Temperature Conversion Chart 45

Vegetable Pita Pizza.. 46

Mushroom Frittata... 47

Sesame Crackers 49

Avocado Smoothie... 50

Roast Pumpkin Soup 51

Homemade Tomato Sauce 52

Crumbed Cashew Fish 54

Prawn Delight.. 56

Salmon and Cantaloupe... 57

Chickpea Tuna Salad... 58

Chili Garlic Shrimp 59

Cranberry Kale Salad 60

Confetti Quinoa Salad 61

Eggplant & Pumpkin Wedges 63

Baked Zucchini Boats 64

Flourless Pizza... 65

Mushroom Cups 67

Crunchy Kale Chips 69

Mashed Cauliflower & Garlic 70

Lemon Pesto.. 71

Fresh Fish Sticks 73

Crockpot Chicken & Bacon 74

Chicken Soup Dinner 76

Hungarian Soup 77

Pork Fajitas 79

BBQ Chicken Wraps 80

Lavender Infused Cutlets 81

Mexican Vegetable Fritters 82

Classic Meatballs 83

Chili Beef 85

Beef & Lemongrass Skewers 86

Beef Stoganoff 88

Crockpot Beef Stew 89

Verde Salsa Beef 90

Hungarian Goulash Crockpot 91

Beef and Vegetable Stir Fry 93

Dijon Pork Chops 94

Pork & Kale Rolls 95

Pumpkin Punch 96

Almond Meal Cookies 97

Raspberry Muffins 99

Fruit Parfait 100

Roasted Rosemary Almonds 101

Other Good Reads 103

Notes 104

.

Introduction

Our addiction to sugar comes at a cost to our health. The onset of diabetes and heart disease are all too common with the foods available to us today. It's possible to prevent the onset of these enemies of society by watching what we eat. **After reading this book you will understand why it is important to lower sugars in your diet and exactly how you can achieve this.** You will learn to identify the pitfalls in modern foods and how to go on and apply this to your everyday life.

Do you want to lose weight, manage your diabetes, lower cholesterol, lower your blood pressure and be full of energy? Dramatically cutting down on sugars in your diet will allow you to succeed. **By eating more natural foods high in nutrition, it will be possible to cut the cravings and feel satisfied with the food you eat.** When you learn to remove harmful high sugar, high carb foods from your diet, and also substitute natural sugar foods in moderation your body will love you for it!

This is the sensible approach to eating sugars, because realistically there will always small amounts of sugar in our diets. By learning where the hidden dangers lie, it is easy to be savvy about it and change our eating habits to make good decisions what we eat. Even some natural foods need to be eaten in moderation, so we'll discuss that too.

This paperback is in black and white print to keep costs down, however if you would like the fully illustrated linked book for Kindle or PC check out my author page on Amazon.

A Wise Chinese Proverb!

"Give a man a fish and you feed him for a day. Teach a man to fish and you feed him for a lifetime." Given this logic, let's learn how to improve our diet and lifestyle long term before we begin with the recipes.

http://www.amazon.com/author/peggy-annear

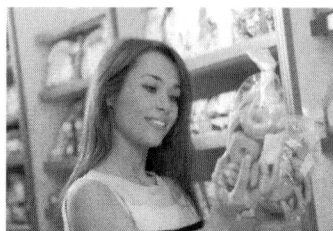

The following pages will teach you **how to identify and tackle problematic sugar issues, which fruits and vegetables are best, which foods to avoid and how to go about eliminating the sugary foods in your diet.** You will learn about total carbs and how to read and understand food labels. The recipes will also point out grams per 100g of sugar and carb content in ingredients that are questionable.

Fructose is a simple sugar that occurs naturally in fruit, vegetables and honey amongst other things. Glucose also naturally occurs in sugar. The more glucose in a food, the more "intestinal friendly" it will be. This applies to all foods including cereals and fruit juices, so read the labels on packaging. The U.S. Nutrition Database search function will also be a helpful tool in helping you to determine how much sugar and other nutrients are in a foods.

How to Remove Sugar from Your Diet!

Start Reading Nutritional Information on Labels!

The American Heart Association advises women limit added sugars to 25 grams (about 6 teaspoons) a day and men to 37.5 grams (about 9 teaspoons) a day. Research also shows that people in Western countries are eating on average about 35 teaspoons of sugar a day! This is because it's hidden in almost all the foods we buy from the supermarket, not straight out of the sugar bowl! We need to take a sensible approach to sugars in our diet.

It's not possible to see added sugars in teaspoons on packaging during manufacturing, but the Nutrition Facts Label can help us to identify added sugars. **Finding ingredients such as sugar, corn syrup,**

dextrose and honey (although honey is at least natural) **near the top of an ingredient list** should signal that there is a high amount of added sugar in the product.

Artificial sweeteners aren't really a healthy long term solution to removing sugar either because of possible adverse health side effects. Stevia and Agave seem to be popular natural plant based sweeteners around right now. However Agave is very high in fructose. But heck, at the end of the day I would rather be eating small amounts of honey, maple syrup or Stevia to my natural foods in moderation as opposed to eating supermarket bought cookies and unhealthy health bars! Some common sense has to come into play. Moderation is key. Don't forget too; homemade biscuits, slices and other recipes can be adapted by reducing sugar and substituting sugar for prunes, maple syrup or dates for example. So if you have the time, it is better to cook your own foods so you know what goes into it! **Your recipes will be free of all those added sugars, additives and preservatives!**

Check Nutritional Information on food labels for Total Carbohydrates as well as Sugars. Carbohydrates are the body's main source of energy. Carbohydrates fall generally into two categories: sugars and starches. Sugar is a simple carbohydrate, and starches, which are complex carbohydrates, break down into blood sugar also known as glucose. **Consuming too many carbohydrates quickly can spike blood sugar levels** which may cause problems over time. Monitoring and maintaining carbohydrate intake is key to blood sugar control. Foods high in sugary carbohydrates include sugary beverages, desserts, dried fruits, sweets, candy, honey and high sugar fruits. Foods high in starchy carbohydrates include starchy vegetables, flour based foods including cereals, peas and beans to a lesser extent, and whole grains such as rice, barley, oats and quinoa. As many of these have high nutritional value, limit them and eat in moderation.

Lignans present in flaxseed, are known to improve the blood sugar levels in type 2 diabetics. Incorporating flaxseed into your meals may be beneficial for you. Ask your doctor or nutritionist. They are readily available from the supermarket.

Start by removing the obvious basic stuff - Remove biscuits, pastries, candy, chocolates and soft drinks from your pantry of fridge.

http://www.amazon.com/author/peggy-annear

Start shopping for more natural foods such as meats, dairy, vegetables, fruit and whole breads. Look for foods unadulterated by processing and manufacturing.

Stop buying hidden high sugar foods that "should" be good for you such as sugary "fruit" muesli, sugary fruit juices and canned fruit, sugary yoghurts and sugary health bars. Cereals can be loaded with sugars or have hidden "clusters" and "dried fruits" that are not natural but rather very sugary.

Look at the labels on foods in your pantry. Your enemies are highly processed foods and condiments such as low fat mayonnaise, tomato ketchup, jam and Hoisin sauce. Some canned meats and soups can be high in sugars. Flavored "juices" and "drinks" are sugar offenders, so check labels.

"Listen" to your taste buds! If something tastes very sweet, it probably has lots of sugar, so investigate further and either eliminate it from your diet altogether, or if it's natural, use in moderation.

Low fat foods usually have more sugar, so check these too. So think about high fibre, low sugar products but beware "lite" products as they usually have lots of sugar. Full cream milk, cream and butter, plus Greek yoghurt and cream cheese are good, eaten in moderation if watching your weight or fat intake of course.

Berries, peaches, pears and kiwi fruit are better for high fibre and lower in sugars than say grapes, bananas and pineapples. But any fresh fruit or vegetable has got to be better than any of the nasty alternatives. Just aim for eating only a few pieces of lower sugar fruits a day is okay.

Homemade salad dressings, such as with olive oil and apple cider vinegar are much better for you than bought brands. Same goes for homemade sauces. If you can make your own with natural ingredients, this is healthier and more nutritious! I regularly make Tzatziki with Greek yoghurt, a little minced garlic and cucumber.

Cut down or remove store bought sugar from cooking, instead substituting with naturally occurring sweet ingredients such as prunes, dates, natural fruit purees, maple syrup and honey. Although these are high is natural sugars, we tend to only use small amounts as a ratio in our meals. Use common sense...No more honey laden toast or pancakes though!

Eggs and Milks: Eggs have hardly any sugar raw; up to around 1g of sugar per 100g depending on how you eat them cooked. Coconut milk has 3.3g of sugar per 100g, cow's milk 5g, and unsweetened almond milk under 1g. So keep these in your diet!

Think about breakfasts: Try an egg on toast, an omelette or a smoothie instead of sugary muffins or pancakes. Maybe some toast with organic peanut butter or cream cheese. Wean yourself off 2 sugars in your coffee or tea! I make up my own low sugar muesli.

Try to cut out the high sugar treats at night time after dinner by substituting the cravings with something else low in sugar such as a glass of unsweetened almond milk (zero sugars and trans fats), raw nuts, celery sticks and dry plain crackers with a very thin slice of cheese and homemade Tzatziki.

Opt for healthy lunches such as sardines, or sliced roast beef or chicken from the supermarket deli section. Team it up with salads, crackers or bread and a piece of fruit. Maybe a smoothie meal in a glass. Once you get some favorites at the supermarket, shopping will be quicker and easier. Remember to read the labels.

Consider looking at the labels on your alcohol, you may be surprised. Liqueurs and sweet wines amongst the culprits to watch.

http://www.amazon.com/author/peggy-annear

What about Honey?

Out with refined sugars, but what about honey? While honey and maple syrup are natural popular substitutes for white processed sugar, they are still high in sugars!

Honey has 82g of sugar per 100g

Maple syrup has 68g sugar per 100g

Let's take the common sense approach. While you will find a few recipes in this book that use these natural sweeteners, it's your choice if you want to remove them altogether or use Stevia or other artificial sweetener instead. My approach is to use the natural foods wherever possible, and **ONLY where you need it for the food to be palatable.** So don't go piling honey on your toast for breakfast because it's natural! Have an egg or avocado instead. It's especially true of people wanting to lose weight but can't stick to a diet that is only meat, salad and veg day in day out.

Of course **an exception to this would be if you can't have any sugars at all due to special dietary conditions.** In this case skip any offending recipes altogether. This is a sugar smart guide to eating foods in a modern world. **This book is designed for a wide range of people, the goal being to help with a better understanding of sugars and how to cut down.**

Bottom line: If you don't want to use honey, skip the recipe altogether!

How to Understand Sugar Amounts on Labels

Locate the "Nutritional Information" on the food packaging. Look for "**Total Carbohydrates**" and "**Sugars**" as both these will be indicated there. (Incidentally, Trans fats are the unhealthy fats) **Remember Fructose and Corn Syrup are some of the worst offenders!** Your goal is to aim for foods lower that 5g if possible. **Analyze the sugar per 100g because per serving varies from product to product.**

Nutrient	Per Serv	Per 100g
Calories (kcal)	130.85	307.7
Calories from Fat (kcal)	28.66	67.39
Fat (g)	3.22	7.58
Saturated Fat (g)	0.61	1.44
Trans Fatty Acid (g)	0.01	0.01
Cholesterol (mg)	0	0
Carbohydrates (g)	21.8	51.27
Dietary Fiber (g)	1.97	4.63
Total Sugars (g)	0.74	1.74
Protein (g)	3.44	8.09
Mono Fat (g)	0.53	1.25

The goal for diabetics, whether or not they use insulin, is to keep their blood sugar as steady as possible and to maximize their intake of nutritious carbs and minimize consumption of less nutritious foods. A starting place for diabetics is to have roughly 45 to 60g of carbs per meal and 15 to 30g for snacks. Consult your doctor.

What is an Acceptable Amount of Sugar?

- **High – over 22g of total sugars per 100g**
- **Low – 5g of total sugars or less per 100g**

*If the amount of sugars per 100g is between these figures, then levels of sugar match accordingly.

*The sugar amount in the nutrition label is the **total amount of sugars in the food**. It includes added sugars and sugars from ingredients such as fruits and milk. Eggs incidentally have around 1g of sugar per 100g (depending if they are cooked) so these are wonderful nutritional packs straight from nature!

Check the Total Carbohydrates

Carbs are the complex part of sugar so they need to be watched as well. For example quinoa may have only 0.9g of sugar per 100g, but has 64g of total carbs! It is also however high in fibre, so this is where a balanced diet full of a variety of natural foods in your best option for health and weight loss. Moderation is the key when eating high carb or high sugar foods. In saying that, all "junk" foods need to be removed altogether as they have virtually no nutritional value whatsoever!

http://www.amazon.com/author/peggy-annear

What is an Acceptable Amount of Carbs?

- **As a guide, if you eat about 2,000 calories a day, you should consume about 250g of complex carbohydrates per day. That is about 1/8th.**

Another example is an average slice of bread. It = approx. 15 grams or 1 serving of carbohydrate.
Although white and wheat bread have very similar carbohydrate content depending on the brands and labels of course, whole-wheat bread is often best. It usually has more than twice the amount of fiber as white bread, meaning you digest it more slowly; hence your blood sugar will rise more gradually after eating it.

Here is an example of a food label that doesn't display sugar per 100g. Always analyze the sugars and total carbs PLUS observe if it's only per Serving Size.

Let's look at the following "health bar" packet. It is high in sugars at 25g and that's not even per 100g but per serving size which is 1 bar! Not healthy, but a way to make it appear that there is less sugar. Also note 33g of total carbohydrates.

Nutrition Facts

Serving Size 1 Bar (85g)
Servings Per Container 4

Amount Per Serving

Calories 170   Calories from Fat 50

	% Daily Value *
Total Fat 6g	9%
Saturated Fat 4g	19%
Trans Fat 0g	
Polyunsaturated Fat 0.5g	
Monounsaturated Fat 1g	
Cholesterol 13mg	4%
Sodium 83mg	3%
Total Carbohydrate 33g	11%
Dietary Fiber 4g	16%
Sugar 25g	
Protein 3g	

Vitamin A 110%   •   Vitamin C 2%
Calcium 10%   •   Iron 3%

*Percent Daily Values are based on a 2,000 calorie diet. Your daily values may be higher or lower depending on your calorie needs.

	Calories	2,000	2,500
Total Fat	Less than	65g	80g
Sat Fat	Less than	20g	25g
Cholesterol	Less than	300mg	300mg
Sodium	Less than	2,400mg	2,400mg
Total Carbohydrate		300g	375g
Dietary Fiber		25g	30g

Calories per gram:
Fat 9   •   Carbohydrate 4   •   Protein 4

The Google Search Method

Do a Google search and discover how much sugar, carbs, fats, protein and calories are in particular foods.

Type into the search bar "how much sugar is in (selected food)"
With some foods you can select from the drop down box under "Type" to narrow your search even further. Similarly, do the same with "how much carbs is in…" See the example below for how much sugar in gm is in 100g banana.

You will also discover the detailed **Nutritional Facts** list from Wikipedia for that particular food on the right hand side of the screen. Try …its an addictive way to look up and learn about food facts quickly!

The Low Sugar Myth

It might be okay in choosing unsweetened milks such as almond milk for example, but you will need to read labels when shopping because low fat products can be loaded with sugars to put some "taste" back in. A classic example of this is in foods such as low fat yoghurts, low fat creams, ice cream and cookies. This from WebMD.com is an interesting read which sums it up well. Sauces and dressings can also be high in sugars which seems surprising. So read labels.

When you read the labels on foods in your supermarket, it's no surprise that you find plenty of sugar in products like cake mix, ice cream, jelly, cookies, and soda. But it can be downright shocking to see 12 grams of sugar in bottled pasta sauce or barbecue sauce -- and even more so to find 50 grams of sugar in a healthy-sounding bottled tea!

To help you ferret out which products are surprisingly high in sugar, I embarked on a mission in the aisles of my local market. Over the course of several days, with my reading glasses close at hand, I examined hundreds of nutrition information labels to check out the sugar content in foods.

One thing's for sure: Just because there's a nutrition-oriented statement on the package (like "contains whole grain," "excellent source of calcium," "fat-free," "100% juice" or "25% less sugar") doesn't mean it *doesn't* contain a shocking amount of sugar. And just because the brand name or product name sounds like it's good for weight loss (Weight Watchers, Skinny Cow, etc.), don't assume the food is lower in sugar.

So how much exactly is a gram of sugar? One teaspoon of granulated sugar equals 4 grams of sugar. To put it another way, 16 grams of sugar in a product is equal to about 4 teaspoons of granulated sugar.

Keep in mind, though, that the grams of sugar listed on the nutrition information label includes natural sugars from fruit (fructose) and milk (lactose) as well as added sweeteners like refined sugar or high-fructose corn syrup. That's why the label on a carton of regular low-fat milk says there's 13 grams of sugar per cup. And that's why the grams of sugar per serving in Raisin Bran (or any cereal with raisins or other dried fruit) seem unexpectedly high.

Also, **carbohydrates are the body's main source of energy and during digestion, sugar which is simple carbohydrates, and starches which are complex carbohydrates, break down into blood sugar also known as glucose.** Consuming too much food that is high in carbohydrates quickly can spike blood sugar levels which may cause problems over time. Monitoring and maintaining carbohydrate intake is key to blood sugar control. **Potato is a classic example. It has under 1g of sugar per 100 g, but has about 20g of carbs.**

http://www.amazon.com/author/peggy-annear

Lentils have about 2g of sugar but 60g of carbs! So does this mean we must never eat potatoes...I'd say heck no unless you have a specific dietary reason. We live in a modern world so just have a few on occasion, not a plate full at once! **Think in terms of balance and moderation.** Talk to your dietician or doctor if you have concerns and want to learn more.

Low Sugar Fruits

Here is a basic guide to low sugar fruits:

-Lemon and Lime
-Rhubarb
-Raspberries
-Blackberries
-Cranberries

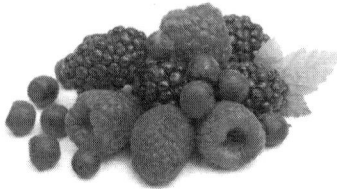

High Sugar Fruits

Eating fruit full of nutrition is better than eating many other high calorie, low nutrient junk foods. However, these fruits should be eaten in moderation.

A Snapshot:

-Tangerines
-Cherries
-Grapes
-Pomegranates
-Mangoes
-Figs
-Bananas
-Dried fruit (raisins, dried apricots, prunes)

Vegetables High in Sugars

Here is a start:

Do the Google Search Method yourself and add to the notes
section below.

Beets - 7g
Carrots - 4.7g. Carrot juice is high in sugars at about 5 gm, while
cooked carrots are low in sugars at about 3 gm.
Corn - 6g
Parsnips - 4.8
Peas - 6g
Potatoes - only about 1.5g of sugar but about 17g of carbs!
Winter Squashes - only around 2g, but about 12g of carbs, especially
acorn and butternut.

Notes

Vegetables Low in Sugar

Alfalfa sprouts
Asparagus
Avocado
Bamboo sprouts
Bean sprouts
Beet greens
Bell pepper (sweet green)
Broccoli
Brussels sprouts
Cabbage -- all kinds
Carrot - Carrot juice is high in sugars (about 5 gm), while cooked carrots are low (about 3 gm).
Cauliflower
Celery
Collard greens
Cucumber
Dandelion greens
Eggplant
Endive
Escarole
Garlic
Green bean, string 3.3g
Kale 1.2g
Leek
Lettuce (all kinds)
Mung bean sprouts
Mushroom
Mustard greens
Okra
Onion
Radish
Arugula
Shallot
Spaghetti squash
Spinach 0.4g
Squash (summer)
Swiss chard

Tomato
Turnip greens
Watercress
Zucchini

Notes

Low Sugar Milks

The Problem with "Light" Products

Beware "fat free" or "light" dairy milks, as they are usually higher in sugars. Stick to full cream dairy milk or natural cream if eating dairy products isn't a concern for you. For weight loss, the following may be helpful.

Unsweetened almond milk has almost no sugar and about 1g of carbs per 100g. Of course different brand stats vary, but almond milk is also popular due to the flavor being pleasant. **It is dairy free and still a good source of calcium.** This is great for people who are lactose intolerant. We drink unsweetened almond milk that is available from the supermarket and it's definitely not too sweet. Rice milk on the other hand is very sweet in flavor and higher in carbs.

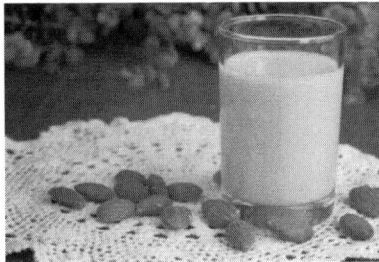

Coconut milk is lower in sugars than dairy milk. Unsweetened coconut milk is available in many supermarkets also. **So there are many options for people who are diabetic, have dairy allergies, or just want to watch their carbohydrate intake for weight loss.** Coconut products are also used in cooking extensively as a dairy free alternative. I love using it in smoothies, baking and curries!

http://www.amazon.com/author/peggy-annear

The Problem with Fructose

Fructose is a problem in the sugar equation. Unfortunately Fructose goes to the liver as fat. The sugar in milk contains glucose and lactose which is deemed to be safe. However honey has about 40% fructose and Agave about 80% which isn't ideal! Some fruits, while generally being healthy and of course far better than candy and junk foods, also have quite a high level of fructose present in them. People suffering with irritable bowel syndrome and other GI disorders may find they are fructose intolerant. Fruits and fruit juices with higher levels of fructose may lead to IBS, abdominal cramping, bloating and diarrhea. So moderation is the key, eating about 1 - 2 pieces a day. Studies have found that eating fruit whole can actually "water down" the effects somewhat due to the water and fibre content. Fresh low fructose fruits and vegetables are best most of the time. Talk to your dietician.

We want to be sensible about it though, because we also understand the beneficial effects on our health and nutrition that fruits and vegetables hold. Berries and kiwi fruits are wonderful natural food sugar treats for weight loss. You can also indulge occasionally on some dark chocolate or similar natural healthy treat.

The American Heart Association recommends that healthy adults strive to eat at least five servings of fruits and vegetables a day to receive the best variety of vitamins, minerals and fiber these foods provide. This is where homemade smoothies and healthy juicer recipes can be helpful. (Check out my Low Sugar Smoothies book over on my author page.)

If you find you aren't getting your daily vitamin allowance through food for some reason, these can help. If possible, fruits and vegetables served whole and/or raw with your meal is best for fibre.

High Fructose Foods

Flavorings that contain fructose are commonly desserts such as ice cream, candy, cookies, "health" bars sweetened with fructose or other sugars. Cereals and other processed foods and junk foods are notorious! If you can't find fructose listed on the food label, here is a general guide (aim for about 10g a day)

Read the Ingredients: Note that **Sugar, Sucrose, Honey, High Fructose Corn Syrup (HFCS) are at least 50% Fructose!**

- Aim for less than 2% sugar – less than 2 grams / 100 grams or ml.
- Compare brands
- Check "low fat dairy" sugar content
- Use Olive Oil, Coconut Oil, Butter and Lard in place of Vegetable oil, Canola oil, Sunflower oil and Margarine, but avoiding Polyunsaturated Oils.

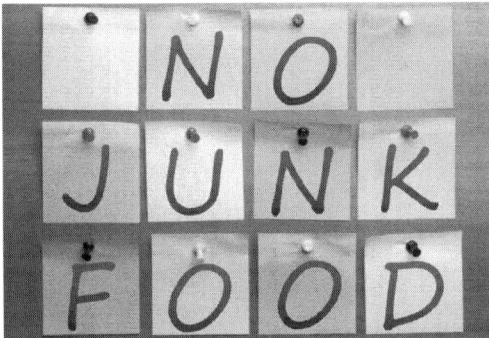

If you have a specific health problem and have been asked by your doctor to eat a low fructose diet, the following is a general guide.

Corn Syrup is made up of almost half glucose and half fructose so should be avoided. It can be found in common food stuffs such as soft drinks, canned, baked or processed foods such as BBQ sauces, jam, ketchup, jellies, chocolate and milks. Again, read labels as varieties will vary in amounts they contain.

http://www.amazon.com/author/peggy-annear

Limit or avoid these high fructose foods where possible. They commonly present digestion and health problems when consumed regularly. Fructose is present in many processed foods so check the labels.

Honey, although high in fructose also happens to be a super food, so this is the natural alternative to sugar I will always go with. **Honey contains over a hundred different compounds, not just fructose and glucose.** It also has small amounts of minerals, amino acids, and vitamins. The point here being...it's not ONLY sugar. **Eat in moderation when a sweetener is needed to make foods palatable.**

Low Fructose Fruits and Vegetables

Here is a list of low fructose ratio fruit and vegetables. They contain about 1% fructose, so are good on the low fructose, higher glucose ratio. These can be eaten as often as you like.

Incidentally, eggs are used in many recipes and they contain around 1g of sugar per 100g, depending on how you eat them.
Apricots (raw)
Avocado
Artichoke
Asparagus
Bean sprouts
Beetroot (fresh)
Broad bean
Brussels sprouts
Broccoli
Cauliflower
Celery
Chinese cabbage
Cranberries
Cucumber
Endives
Grapefruit
Ginger
Green beans
Green capsicum

Green chili
Green pea
Kale
Limes
Lemons
Lettuce
Mushroom
Parsley
Parsnip
Potato
Pumpkin
Radish
Rhubarb
Silverbeet
Snow pea
Spinach
Sweetcorn
Tamarillo
Watercress
Zucchini

Moderate Fructose Fruits & Vegetables

Here is a list of low fructose ratio fruit and vegetables. They contain about 2 % fructose which is still quite low, so are good on the low fructose, higher glucose ratio too.

Apricots (canned)
Beetroot (canned)
Banana capsicum
Blackcurrants
Chives
Cabbage
Carrots
Eggplant
Fennel
Grapefruit
Guava (raw)
Honeydew melon

Green olives
Marrow
Mulberry
Nectarines
Orange
Pineapple (raw)
Raspberries
Passion fruit (fresh/tinned)
Peaches (fresh or tinned)
Plums
Red capsicum
Red chili
Squash
Swede
Sweet potato
Shallot
Strawberries
Tangelos
Turnip
Tomato (raw)
Turnip
Watermelon

High Fructose Fruits

High fructose fruits that have up to about 5 % fructose on the low fructose, higher glucose ratio. When starting a low fructose diet, this group should be avoided. Once problematic symptoms settle down you can then **eat only small amounts from this group.**

Banana
Blackberry (raw/frozen)
Cherries (raw)
Figs (raw)
Kiwi fruit
Mandarin (canned in syrup)
Mandarin
Mango
Paw paw

Pineapple (canned in natural juice)
Rock melon
Star fruit

Very High Fructose Ratio

This is a list of very high fructose fruits; that is over 5%.

Apple
Blueberries (frozen/fresh)
Canned dark plums **in syrup**
Custard apple
Canned fruits **in syrup** (berries, cherries, raspberries, strawberries, blueberries)
Dried fruit (figs, apricots, dates, prunes, sultanas, raisins, currants)
Gherkins
Grapes
Lychee
Nashi pear
Pear
Persimmon
Pickled onion
Pomegranate
Quince
Tomato paste (and similar products)

Remember though...it's generally better for your health to pick up an apple or a banana than junk foods!

http://www.amazon.com/author/peggy-annear

Variety is Key

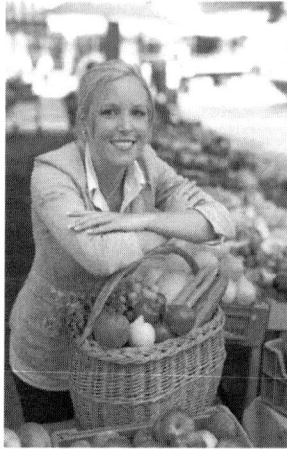

For most people, eating a mixed variety of vegetables and fruits following the low sugar guidelines will help control your sugar intake. Our modern day society laced with Fructose can effect and be the cause of diabetes, bad cholesterol and heart problems. It really is like the sweet poison.

Supermarket foods laced with preservatives, additives, chemicals and high carbohydrates often have little nutritional value, so going fresh, natural is best. Healthy snacks such as low fructose vegetables, raw cocao, home made treats mixed with some olive or coconut oil, seeds and nuts (especially raw almonds) are all fine.

The U.S. Nutrition Database may be helpful to do a further search.

The French Connection

Digestion and the auto immune system can also be effected by loading your body with sugars. So if you are constantly having tummy problems or bloating, then this may be the cause. Try removing sugars from your diet for even just a few days and see if you notice any change.

The French are renowned for replacing sugar in their diet with fat and protein, and it seems to work! This is why the Paleo lifestyle eating plan is so popular. So if you think you are eating healthy by buying that low fat dairy product, don't do it because it is probably replaced with just more sugars! Also be aware that many supermarket foods are laced with sugars that you wouldn't think possible. For example how could ketchup be sugary you might ask...well it is. Read the labels, if it's got high amounts of sugars and Fructose disguised in it, stay clear.

Let's get started with some recipes!

I've tried to add sugar and carb counts where they may be questionable. If you get stuck, refer back to the Google Search Method I gave you earlier.

Omit or add ingredients where it makes sense for you. Remember to buy fresh, unprocessed natural foods where possible.

Nut & Seed Granola

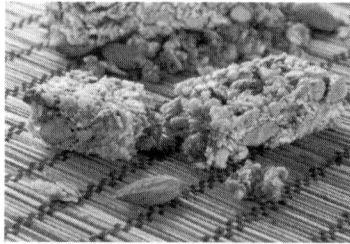

These make great snacks or treats but if you feel like some primal crunch for breakfast – crush some up into a bowl and add some cold unsweetened almond milk for a terrific treat!

Ingredients:

- 3 cups assorted nuts & seeds (almonds 4g sugar, walnuts 2.6g, sunflower seeds 2.6g, etc)

- 1/4 cup fresh cranberries (fresh has 4g sugar, dried has about 65g)

- 2 cups shredded coconut (unsweetened)

- ¼ cup coconut oil

- ½ cup sunflower seed butter

- ½ cup honey or maple syrup (honey has 82g of sugar per 100g, maple syrup has 68g sugar per 100g)

- ¼ tsp vanilla extract, optional (13g of sugar per 100g)

- ½ tsp salt

- 1 tsp cinnamon

- 1 Tbsp chia seeds

Directions:

1. Line a baking dish or tray with baking paper and set aside.
2. Combine nuts and seeds into large bowl.
3. Remove 1 cup of nuts & seeds mix and chop into small pieces.
4. Place remaining 2 cups of nuts & seeds in blender and pulse till chopped quite finely – You should end up with a good mix of small and fine pieces.
5. Return nuts & seeds to mixing bowl. Stir in dried cranberries and add coconut. Stir well combining contents together.
6. Place a small saucepan on a low-med flame and add coconut oil, sunflower seed butter & honey, vanilla, salt & cinnamon to cook. Stir until mixture bubbles and then remove from heat.
7. Pour hot liquid mixture over nut mixture, stirring to combine. Add chia seed if you haven't already. Mix well.
8. Pour the combined nuts-and-honey mixture into prepared tray and press together using wet hands or spoon pressing firmly to ensure ingredients are well packed together.
9. Leave mixture to sit for 2 hours, cover and then place in freezer for at least 1 hour.
10. Remove from freezer and cut into chunk sized pieces or muesli bars slices with a very sharp knife. You can eat like this or serve crumbled up for a grain free

Apricot Smoothie

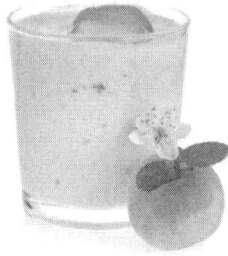

Unsweetened almond milk works in this recipe instead of yoghurt if you are weight watching. However the flavor won't be as rich and texture not as creamy.

Ingredients:

- •1 cup raw halved apricots

- •6 ice cubes

- •1 cup plain natural yogurt

- •1 Tbsp honey or equivalent Stevia sweetener (optional)

Directions:

1. Blend apricots, yogurt, ice cubes & sugar in a blender until mixture is thick and frothy. (serves 2)

*Packs a sweet-n-sour tang that's extra refreshing. Place an apricot half on top if desired.

Savory French Toast

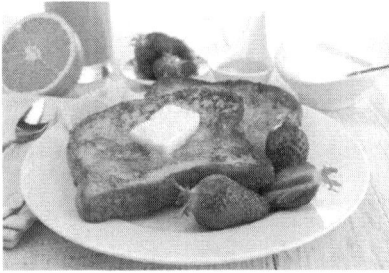

Google the list of sugars and carbs in common breads. Whole grain is best. (Search with the drop down box.)

Ingredients:

- oil for frying

- 2 slices whole grain, high fibre low carb breads

- ¼ cup milk

- 3 eggs

- 1 tsp mixed dried herbs

- salt & pepper to taste

- dob of cream cheese on top (optional)

Directions:

1. Toast the bread.
2. Mix the eggs, milk, seasonings and herbs using a fork in a flat pie plate (large enough to lay toast in).
3. Warm the oil in a skillet on medium heat.
4. Dip the toast in the egg mix, then fry it on the skillet for 2 minutes on each side until golden.
   Serve with cream cheese, berries or eat as it is.

Apple Pie Oatmeal

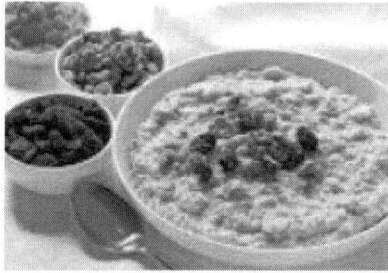

Oats is low in sugar and low in GI making it good for a satisfying breakfast. It is high in carbs but fibre too. So eat in moderation. Raisins are okay if you want an occasional treat. Just only use a small amount as they have 59g of sugar per 100g! I use prunes, chopped. They are an excellent source of fibre and come in at 38g of sugar.

Ingredients:

- 1 cup milk (unsweetened almond works too)

- ½ cup oatmeal (oatmeal have has 0.5g sugar per 100g and 12g of carbs)

- ¼ cup unsweetened applesauce or homemade stewed apricots to keep sugar down.

- 1 tsp prunes, chopped

- ½ tsp vanilla

- ¼ tsp cinnamon

- ¼ tsp nutmeg

Directions:

1. Cook the oats in milk. Once they are done add applesauce and prunes, as well as vanilla, cinnamon and nutmeg.
2. Decorate with walnuts or other roasted nuts.

Almond Flour Crepes

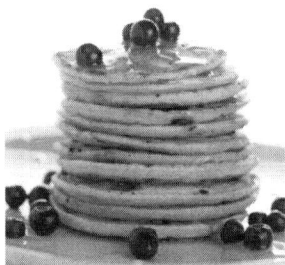

Almond flour is low in sugar and carbs

Ingredients:

- 1½ cups almond flour (2g of sugar per 100g and about 12g of carbs per 1/2 cup)

- 1 cup of milk (½ cup for thicker pancakes. Milk has 5g of sugar per 100g)

- 3 eggs

- ½ cup strawberries or blueberries

- spices by your choice such as cinnamon, vanilla, nutmeg or others

- oil for cooking (olive oil is good)

Directions:

1. Combine all ingredients except blueberries in a small bowl. Blend them with a blender until the batter is smooth.
2. Mix in the blueberries.
3. Warm the oil in a frying pan.
4. Cook all pancakes. It should take about 2-3 minutes for each side to get golden brown.
5. Serve and enjoy!

Kale Smoothie Blend

Have this smoothie for breakfast, lunch or when you are on the run! This recipe is inspired from the allergy free, natural foods**, Lunch Box Recipes book by Jane Burton on Amazon**. They suggest you can also freeze it in a bottle and put it a lunchbox and/or take it to work.

Ingredients:

- 1 cup fresh kale or baby spinach, washed

- 1 cup strawberries (for sweetness)

- 1/2 avocado, peeled, de-seeded and chopped

- juice from 1/2 a lemon or lime

- 2 - 3 kiwifruit, peeled and chopped (for sweetness)

*Can add 1 tsp chia seeds and 1 tsp flaxseed oil for extra goodness.

Directions:

1. Process all ingredients in a blender until well mixed.
2. Pour into glasses and garnish if desired with a slice of strawberry.

Eggnog

Ingredients:

- 1 cup full cream or unsweetened almond milk (cream has about 2g of sugar per 100gm and 2 g of carbs. Unsweetened almond milk has almost no sugar and about 1g of carbs per 100g)

- 1 large egg

- 1/2 tsp cinnamon

- 1/2 tsp nutmeg

- 1/4 tsp vanilla extract

- dash of rum (optional)

Directions:

1. Blend all ingredients. Pour the smoothie into glasses topped with a sprinkle of cinnamon or sliced fruit. Serve and enjoy!

Vegetable V8 Drink

A nutritious meal in a glass!

Ingredients:

- ½ cup tomato, chopped

- ½ cup ice

- ¼ cup cucumber, chopped

- ¼ cup raw spinach

- ½ avocado

- 2 tsp fresh lemon juice

- 1 tsp Tabasco (optional)

Directions:

1. Blend all ingredients and the ice until smooth. Avocado is the main source of energy in this recipe, while other ingredients provide vitamins and, of course, great taste.

Lunch Smoothie

Inspired from my **Low Sugar Smoothies** book.

Ingredients:

- 1 ripe pear - (cored & cut into chunk size pieces)

- 1 cup freshly squeezed orange juice

- 1-2 cups washed spinach leaves

- 1 cup broccoli florets - (lightly steamed to reduce hardness)

- 1 cup strawberries

- 1 cup natural yogurt

Directions:

1. Place all ingredients in a blender and puree until smooth. Serve immediately. The combination of green veggies and fresh fruit for lots of health promoting goodness!

Oven Temperature Conversion Chart

Table of equivalent oven temperatures[1]		
Description	°C	°F
Cool oven	90°C	200°F
Very Slow oven	120°C	250°F
Slow oven	150–160°C	300–325°F
Moderately Slow	160–180°C	325–350°F
Moderate oven	180–190°C	350–375°F
Moderately Hot	190–200°C	375–400°F
Hot oven	200–230°C	400–450°F
Very Hot oven	230–260°C	450–500°F
Fast oven	230–260°C	450–500°F

Vegetable Pita Pizza

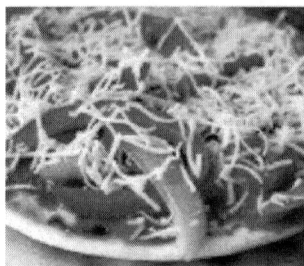

Ingredients:

- 1 whole low carb pita bread of your choice

- ½ cup mixed sliced vegetables of your choice (I like onion, baby spinach, basil, sun dried tomato and olive)

- ¼ cup tomato canned or cooked homemade tomato ketchup (canned have about 2.5g sugar, supermarket tomato sauce is around 22g sugar!)

- ¼ cup cheese of your choice, grated (can't beat a little Parmesan at 1g sugar and 4.1g of carbs)

- cooking spray for coating

Directions:

Preheat the oven to 450°F (230°C).

1. Use the cooking spray on a baking sheet. Place the pita bread on it.
2. Spread the tomato sauce on pita bread. Top with vegetables of your choice. Sprinkle the cheese over.
3. Bake for 8 minutes or until cheese is lightly brown.

*Check common flour statistics for sugar and carbs by doing the Google Search Method.

Mushroom Frittata

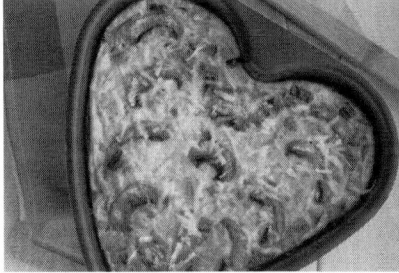

Ingredients:

- 8 eggs, beaten

- 8 oz (225g) mushrooms, sliced

- 5 oz (140g) chicken breast or bacon pieces, cooked and diced

- 1 green bell pepper, chopped

- ½ low carb flour or 1/3 cup of whole grain flour

- 1 Tbsp flaxseed (optional)

- ½ cup feta cheese, chopped

- 1 tsp baking powder

- salt and black pepper to taste

Cooking spray for coating

Directions:

Preheat the oven to 400°F (200°C).

1. In a frying pan sauté the mushrooms and bell pepper for about 3 minutes on high heat. Reduce the heat to medium and cook for one more minute.
2. In a bowl mix the eggs with flour baking powder, flaxseed, salt and pepper. Stir in almost all of the cheese.
3. Combine the crumbled patties with mushrooms and bell pepper. You can do it in the same pan.
4. Coat a baking dish with cooking spray. Place the mushroom, bell pepper and meat mixture in it. Pour the egg mixture over. If you wish you can add some mushroom slices on top or sprinkle the frittata with some more cheese.
5. Bake for 40 minutes in the oven or until done. Cut the fritatta in squares.

Sesame Crackers

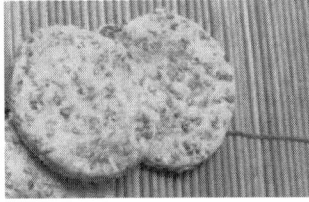

Almond flour is nutritious, low in sugar and carbs compared to other flours.

Ingredients:

- 3 cups almond meal flour (2g of sugar per 100g and about 12g of carbs per 1/2 cup)

- 1 cup sesame seeds

- 1/4 cup poppy seeds (optional)

- 2 eggs, whisked

- 2 Tbsp olive oil

- 1½ tsp salt

Directions:

1. Preheat the oven to 350° F (180°C).
2. Mix all ingredients in a big bowl.
3. Line two large baking sheets with parchment paper. Place half of the dough right in the middle of each sheet. Place another piece of parchment paper over the dough mounds.
4. Evenly roll the dough between the parchment papers until it covers entire baking sheet. Do for both baking sheets. Remove parchment paper and cut the dough with a scone circular cutter, or by hand with a knife. You can also use a glass.

Bake for 10-15 minutes or until golden brown.

http://www.amazon.com/author/peggy-annear

Avocado Smoothie

Avocados are low in sugar and loaded with healthy oils and nutrition. This is great if you don't feel like a particularly sweet smoothie drink.

Ingredients:

- 1 ripe avocado (0.7g of sugar per 100g and 9g of carbs)

- 1 cup unsweetened almond milk (almost nil sugar and 1g of carbs)

- 2 tsp honey or Stevia equivalent (optional)

- 1 basil leaf

- squeeze of lime juice

Directions:

Place milk in blender, then all other ingredients and mix well. Serve chilled. Add a sprig of parsley or basil on top.

Roast Pumpkin Soup

Ingredients:

- 2kg (4 1/2 pounds) approximately of pumpkin (pumpkin has 2.8g of sugar per 100g and 6g of carbs)

- 2 Tbsp olive oil

- 4 cups home made chicken stock with bone

- 1 1/2 cups water

- salt and ground black pepper

- ½ tsp onion or garlic flakes

- 1 tsp dried tarragon leaves

- pinch of mild curry powder (optional, but tasty!)

Directions:

1. Prepare pumpkin by cutting in half and removing the seeds. Brush with oil; placing onto baking sheet in hot oven (350F); cut side facing down and bake for about 1 hour or until done.
2. When cooked, scoop out pumpkin flesh with a spoon and place into a large cooking pot. Add stock and water. Add garlic flakes, tarragon leaves, curry powder and seasonings, mix well with hand held stick blender until smooth.
3. Place pot on a medium to high heat and bring to the boil. Reduce heat to very low and simmer for about 1 hour; stirring occasionally. (Add 1/4 cup cream cheese at this point if desired)
4. Blend once slightly cooled and re heat if required.

Homemade Tomato Sauce

You can double this recipe up!

Ingredients:

- 1 Tbsp olive oil

- 2 garlic cloves minced

- 1 cup chopped onion

- ¼ cup apple cider vinegar (about 4g of sugar per 100g)

- ¼ cup red wine vinegar (Nil sugar)

- ¼ cup honey or Stevia alternative (85g of sugar per 100gm is high, but it is at least natural. Use Stevia sweetening if desired)

- 1 tsp salt

- 28 ounce can tomato puree (canned tomatoes have about 2.5g sugar per 100g)

- half a 12 ounce can tomato paste (tomato paste has about 11g sugar per 100g, so we aren't using much)

- ½ tsp ground cloves

- ½ tsp oregano

Directions:

1. Heat the oil and sauté garlic for a few minutes.
2. Add the onion and cook for 3 minutes until softened.
3. Mix in the vinegars, salt and honey.
4. Add tomato paste and puree, bringing to the boil.
5. Now mix in the oregano and the cloves.
6. Reduce the sauce so it thickens, for about 15 minutes.

7. Blend until smooth.

    *Place into air tight jars in the fridge, or freeze some in plastic containers.

Crumbed Cashew Fish

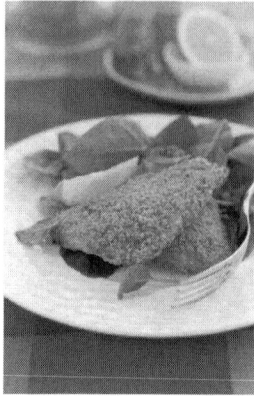

Cashews have 6g of sugar per 100g and 30g of carbs. However, remember they are packed with vitamins, protein and fibre and only eaten in moderation.

Ingredients:

- 400g (14oz) white fish (cut into palm sized pieces)

- 2 tsp coriander

- 2 tsp cumin

- 2 tsp black peppercorns

- 2 tsp black mustard seed

- 3 Tbsp cashew nut meal flour

- A pinch cayenne pepper

- A handful of crushed cashews (6g of sugar per 100g)

- 1 onion peeled & finely chopped

- Olive oil

- A handful of fresh coriander or parsley

Directions:

1. Grind black peppercorns and mustard seeds with mortar & pestle.
2. Combine ground pepper, mustard, cumin, coriander & cayenne in a bowl. Add cashew flour.
   Heat a frypan to high, dry fry crushed cashews till golden and then set aside.
3. Add small amount of oil to pan; sauté onions for 5 minutes and then set aside with cashews.
4. Add enough oil to frypan to shallow fry fish which has been generously coated with cashew and spice mix. Fish should only need about 2-3 minutes each side. Fry till crisp and golden!
5. Return onions and cashews to frypan for 1- 2 minutes adding seasoning.
6. Serve with fresh coriander and a handful of baby spinach leaves.

Prawn Delight

Ingredients:

- 4 tsp olive oil

- 500g med raw prawns (shrimp has nil sugar and 1.5g of carbs)

- 6-8 minced garlic cloves

- 1 cup chicken stock

- ¼ cup fresh lemon juice

- ¼ cup and 1 tbsp extra minced parsley

- Salt and pepper

- 4 lemon wedges (lemon has 2.5g of sugar per 100g)

Directions:

1. Heat oil in large frypan. Sauté prawns over low-med heat till pink; approx. 2-3 minutes.
2. Add garlic. Cook stirring constantly for 30 seconds. Transfer prawns to a dish / platter. Cover & keep prawns warm in very low oven.
3. Combine chicken stock, lemon juice, wine ¼ cup of the parsley & seasonings in frypan; and bring to boil.
4. Continue boiling until sauce is reduced by half.
   Spoon sauce over prawns; garnish with lemon and sprinkle remaining tbsp parsley. Serve with freshly made salad greens.

Salmon and Cantaloupe

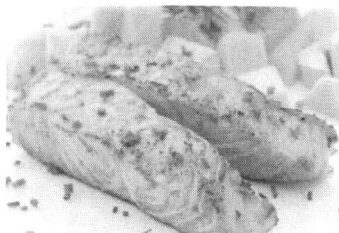

Ingredients:

- about 1 pound or 500g salmon fillets

- salt and pepper to taste

- 1 medium lemon, sliced

- 1/2 Cantaloupe, peeled, de-seeded and chopped (8g sugar per 100g and 8g of carbs)

- 1 Tbsp olive oil

Directions:

1. Place salmon fillets skin side down on baking sheet lined with foil.
2. Season with salt and pepper
3. Place sliced lemons and chopped cantaloupe over salmon
4. Drizzle lightly with olive oil
5. Cover with cling plastic; placing in fridge for 1- 2 hours
6. Bake salmon meal in medium - hot (400F/205C) oven for 12- 15 minutes
7. Serve with fresh steamed vegetables or a side salad.

Chickpea Tuna Salad

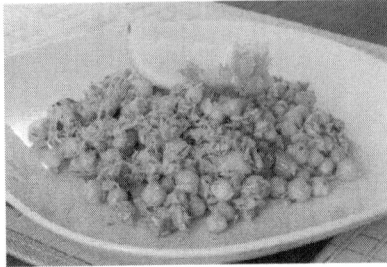

Chickpeas are **nutritious but high in carbs, so eat in moderation.**

Ingredients:

- 2 cups chickpeas (cooked chickpeas have 4.8g of sugar per 100g, but 27g of carbs)

- 2 cups tuna

- 3 big stalks green onion, chopped

- 1 Tbsp olive oil

- ½ Tbsp lemon juice

- salt and black pepper to taste

Directions:

1. Combine chickpeas, tuna and onion in a salad bowl. Sprinkle with olive oil and lemon juice. Add salt and black pepper to taste. Mix well.
2. This salad can be served on its own or on a slice of bread or plain crackers. Enjoy!

Chili Garlic Shrimp

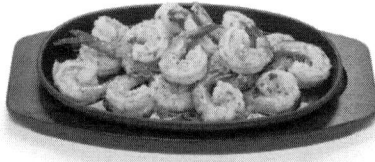

Ingredients:

- ½ pound, about 225g raw shrimp (prawns) peeled (shrimp has nil sugar and 1.5g of carbs)

- 6 cloves garlic, minced

- 2 Tbsp olive oil (can also use olive oil)

- 1/2 Tbsp chili powder

- ½ Tbsp parsley

- salt, black pepper to taste

Directions:

1. Heat olive oil in a pan over medium-high heat.
2. When the oil is hot, fry shrimp for 1 minute.
3. Add chili powder, garlic, parsley and cayenne pepper and cook for 5 more minutes.
4. Serve with rice or quinoa and enjoy!

Cranberry Kale Salad

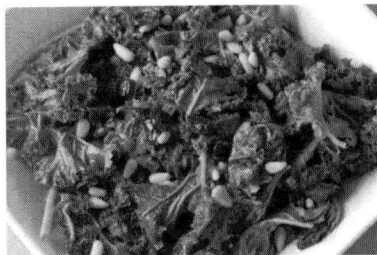

Very flexible with vegetable ingredients, so experiment with things like grated carrot, red cabbage, baby spinach leaves and salad onion - use what you have on hand!

Ingredients:

- 1 cup chopped kale of your choice

- 1/2 cup fresh whole or halved cranberries (4g of sugar per 100g and 12g of carbs)

- 1 Tbsp pine nuts or walnuts (if desired, toast pine nuts first as this gives a nice flavor)

- 1 Tbsp melted butter or maple syrup (about 67g of sugar and carbs per 100g are in maple syrup)

- 1 Tbsp olive oil

- 1/2 Tbsp freshly squeezed lemon juice

Directions:

1. Chop the kale finely, or break into small pieces.
2. Transfer to a salad bowl. Add the cranberries and nuts.
3. Mix the honey, olive oil and lemon juice together in a cup. Toss all together.

Confetti Quinoa Salad

Quinoa makes a filling and nutritious meal on occasion. It is a good alternative to potato, **but is high in carbs, so only eat in moderation.** Play around with the ingredients. Sometimes dried apricot is nice for a change. This salad has been added because it has loads of nutrition in it.

Ingredients:

- 3/4 cup water

- 1 tsp olive oil

- 1/2 cup quinoa, uncooked and rinsed (under 1g of sugar per 100g but 64g of carbs)

- 1/2 red onion, finely chopped (spring onions work too)

- 1/4 cup green and/or red capsicum pepper, diced (Red has 4.3g of sugar per 100g and 7g of carbs. Green has 2.4g of sugar and 2.4g of carbs)

- 1/4 tsp mild curry powder

- juice of 1/2 a lemon

- 1/2 cup mixed diced vegetables such as kale, carrot and green beans

- about 1 - 2 Tbsp of chopped fresh herbs such as basil, parsley, chives or cilantro

- salt and ground black pepper to taste

- 1 chopped avocado

- a handful of cherry tomatoes and baby spinach (optional - when serving)

Directions:

1. Cook the quinoa as per directions: bring water to the boil and pour in quinoa and oil. Reduce heat to a simmer and boil for about 15 mins or until water has been absorbed.
2. Place the cooked quinoa into a bowl, and chill in refrigerator until cold, around 20 mins.
3. Remove quinoa from fridge and stir in all the other ingredients except avocado and tomato.
4. Season to taste with salt and pepper.
5. Chill before freezing.

Eggplant & Pumpkin Wedges

Can use Pumpkin or Eggplant in this recipe. Eggplant doesn't take as long to cook! Eat these veggies in moderation.

Ingredients:

- 2 cups pumpkin, cut into 3/4 inch wedges (pumpkin has 2.3g sugar to 100g and 4.9g carbs. Eggplant has 3.2g of sugar and 9g of carbs)

- about 1/2 cup olive oil for cooking

- 1 cup all purpose plain flour, on a plate

- 1 tsp salt

- 1 tsp ground black pepper

- 1 tsp dried mixed herbs

*For a garnish twist you can sprinkle this dish with ground nuts, coconut or some dried herbs!

Directions:

1. After slicing the pumpkin, place in a bowl of water and soak for 1 hour.
2. Remove pumpkin from the water, allow excess water to drip off.
3. Toss in the flour. Shake off excess.
4. Fry over medium heat in some oil. Do in batches, turning till golden brown.

*Serve in a bowl with garnish or dip if desired.

http://www.amazon.com/author/peggy-annear

Baked Zucchini Boats

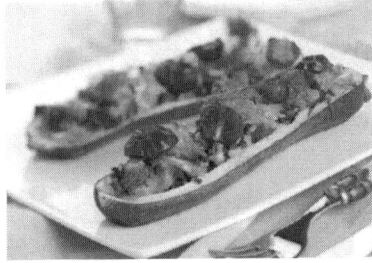

Ingredients:

The cooking time will depend on the size of your zucchinis...big boats for luncheons, or little boats as a side meal. Mushrooms work well chopped up in this also.

- 1 Tbsp olive oil

- 1 pound or about 500gm lean minced beef (can use bacon pieces)

- 1 large chopped brown onion

- 3 - 4 chopped cloves garlic

- 2 fat zucchinis, seeded and cut in half lengthways(1.7g of sugar per 100g and 2.7g of carbs)

- 6 tsp tomato puree from a can (can use halved fresh tomato. Canned tomato has 2.4g sugar per 100g, fresh red tomato has 2.6g of sugar)

- 1/2 Tbsp white vinegar (nil g of sugar)

- 1/2 cup chopped parsley or chives

- 1/4 tsp of ground black pepper

- 2 Tbsp toasted pine nuts or walnuts (optional. Pine nuts have 3.6g of sugar per 100g, walnuts 2.6g)

Directions:

Preheat the oven to 350°F (180°C).

1. Prepare the zucchini and place on a foil lined oven tray.
2. Combine the tomato and vinegar in a cup. Set aside.
3. Heat a pan to high and quickly brown the onion, mince and finally the garlic in the oil (don't over cook)
4. Add the herbs and scrape the mixture out into the zucchini boats. Pour the tomato puree over the top.
5. Cook in the oven for about 20 mins covered with foil, then uncovered for another 10 mins. (The slow cooker can be used for this dish as another cooking option)
Serve on a platter as a side meal, or for lunch.

Flourless Pizza

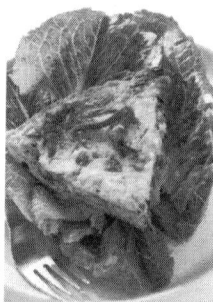

Don't over load with toppings otherwise it will take longer to cook properly. We like mushrooms, bok choy or spinach, tomato, onion, bell pepper and garlic.

Ingredients:

- 7 eggs

- 6 oz full fat cream cheese, softened (cream cheese has about 3g of sugar and 4.1g carbs. Low fat has 6g of sugar and 8g of carbs)

- 1 tsp garlic powder

- ½ tsp salt

- 1½ tsp dried Marjoram or Oregano

- a pinch of black pepper

- a pinch of cayenne pepper

- 1 cup of grated Parmesan (Parmesan has 1g sugar per 100g and 4.1g of carbs)

Directions:

Heat the oven to 350°F (180°C).

1. Make sure cream cheese is at room temperature.
2. Mix the egg and cream cheese in a blender or food processor until well blended.
3. Add the salt and spices and blend again.
4. Spread the Parmesan cheese in the bottom of a well greased 9X13 pan.
5. Pour the egg mixture over the cheese, and bake for 22-25 minutes, or until the top is golden brown.
6. Remove from the oven, add your preferred pizza toppings, and bake for about 10 - 15 more minutes until done.

Mushroom Cups

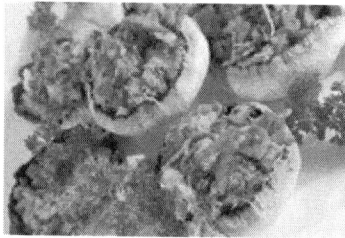

Ingredients:

- about 10 - 15 small to medium sized fresh mushrooms

- oil to cook bacon

- 2 rashers of bacon strips, diced

- 1/2 cup diced spring onions

- 1 clove garlic, minced or diced

- 1/2 cup grated Parmesan cheese (0.9 of sugar per 100g and 4.1 of carbs)

- 1 fresh tomato or 1 cup eggplant, diced

- 1/2 small zucchini, diced (2.5g of sugar per 100g and 3.1 of carbs)

- 1/2 tsp ground black pepper

- 1/2 tsp salt or to taste

*Using sardines and olives instead of bacon gives this dish a distinct Provencal twist.

http://www.amazon.com/author/peggy-annear

Directions:

1. Remove stems from the mushrooms, setting the caps aside. Dice the stems.
   In a pan with oil cook the bacon over medium heat until crisp. Add the mushroom stems cooking for a minute.
2. Drain on paper towels. Remove from the heat.
3. Stir in the remaining ingredients.
4. Firmly stuff the mixture into the mushroom caps, but don't overfill. Place in a greased 15 in. x 10-in. x 1 in. baking pan or similar tray.
5. Bake in a hot oven at 425 for 10 - 15 minutes or until mushrooms are tender, depending on their size. Garnish with fresh herbs.

Crunchy Kale Chips

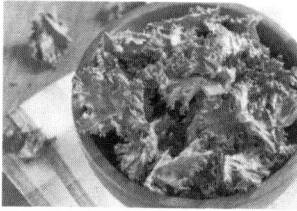

A good alternative to potato chips!

Ingredients:

- a bunch of kale, broken into even sized pieces (1.2g of sugar per 100g and 9g of carbs)

- oil by your choice (olive, coconut or any other oil with mild taste)

- 1 tsp salt

- seasoning of your choice (such as garlic, dried bell pepper, chili, thyme, curry, dried basil etc)

Directions:

Preheat the oven to 300°F (150°C).

1. Cover a baking sheet with parchment paper.
2. Tear the kale leaves in evenly chip-sized pieces. If the sizes vary a lot, it is very likely that some chips will get burnt while others aren't done yet.
3. In a bowl mix these pieces thoroughly with the oil, salt and seasoning, then place them on the covered baking sheet.
4. Be very careful not to burn the chips. It usually takes 5 to 10 minutes for the kale chip sides to get brown and ready to serve.

Mashed Cauliflower & Garlic

A good alternative to high carb potato.

Ingredients:

- 1 large cauliflower (most of the core removed) cut into florets
- 1 Tbsp natural butter
- 1 tsp salt
- 1/2 tsp ground black pepper to taste
- 1 tsp garlic flakes or fresh garlic (optional)
- 2 Tbsp full cream
- fresh or dried mixed herbs (optional - depending on what you are serving it with)

Directions:

1. Prepare cauliflower and cut into florets. Place in a double steamer saucepan and steam until almost done. You can boil the cauliflower if you don't have a steamer, but steaming holds more of the nutrients and flavor.
2. Tip cauliflower into a glass bowl or food processor once slightly cooled and add all the other ingredients. Mash by hand or process together until smooth. Garnish with herbs if desired.

Lemon Pesto

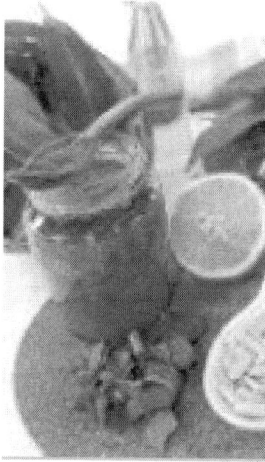

This is an extravagant sauce for special treats.

Ingredients:

- juice and zest of 1 lemon

- 1 cup fresh basil leaves

- 3/4 cup baby spinach leaves (nil sugar and 3.6g of carbs)

- 1/4 cup of olive oil

- 1/4 cup of toasted pine nuts(3.6g of sugar and 13g of carbs)

- 1/4 cup of toasted salted cashews (6g of sugar per 100g and 30g of carbs)

- 1 clove of garlic

- salt and pepper to taste

Directions:

*Toast the nuts by heating a dry tray to medium heat on the stove top, turning the nuts constantly for a few mins. so you don't burn them.

1. Zest the lemon and remove 2 Tbsp of the juice.
2. Place all the ingredients together into a food processor or blender and blend into a course mix. Smooth is okay if you prefer.

* Another appetizer accompaniment favorite, just store in the refrigerator for up to one day.

Fresh Fish Sticks

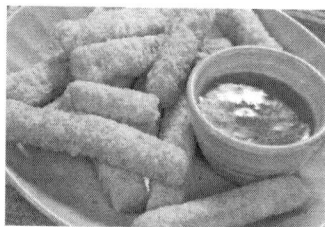

Ingredients:

- 1 pound or about 450g white fresh fish fillets (for example, tilapia, cod, whiting or snapper)

- 2 eggs, whisked

- 1 cup low carb flour, or almond flour

- olive oil for frying

- salt to taste

  Use a dipping sauce of your choice, or lemon wedges.

Directions:

1. Rinse fish fillets and cut them in finger sized sticks (1x4 inches or 2x10cm), removing fish bones on the way.
2. Heat the olive oil in a big skillet on medium high heat.
3. Prepare two bowls: one with egg and other with almond flour and salt.
4. Dip the fish sticks first in egg, then almond flour and place on the skillet.
5. Cook on each side for 2-3 minutes until well browned. Repeat the process as necessary.
6. Serve at a picnic lunch or a TV dinner with a homemade sauce or lemon wedges.

Crockpot Chicken & Bacon

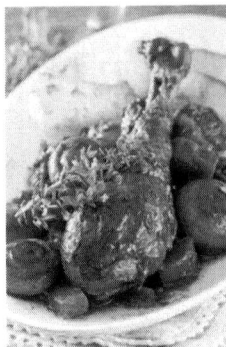

Ingredients:

- 3 Tbsp olive oil

- 5 - 6 chicken pieces (with excess fat and skin removed)

- 5 lean rashers of bacon, diced (nil sugar, nil carbs)

- 2 brown onions

- 1 chopped garlic clove

- 1/2 cup chopped, halved mushrooms

- 1/4 cup low carb flour

- 1 cup homemade chicken stock

- 1 1/2 cups dry red wine (about 0.5g of sugar for 100g and about 2g of carbs. Dry is better than sweet)

- 2 bay leaves

- 1/2 tsp mixed herbs

- salt to taste

- black pepper to taste, ground

Directions:

1. Heat a heavy based pan to medium high and brown all the chicken in the oil. Transfer into the crock pot.
2. In the same pan, fry the bacon and onions for about 3 minutes till partially crispy and browned.
3. Stir in the garlic and mushrooms for about 5 minutes more.
4. Now blend in the flour, again cooking for about 2 - 3 minutes, then gradually blend in the stock and wine.
5. Place all this mix into the crock pot and add the bay leaves, herbs and seasonings.
6. Cook on low for about 6 hours or high for about 4.

Chicken Soup Dinner

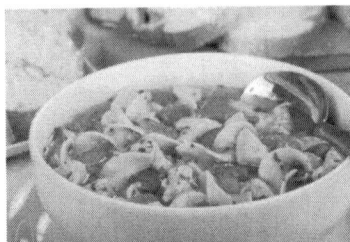

This is a low sugar, healthy meal coming in at around 1.6g of sugar per 100g. Leave out noodles if desired.

Ingredients:

- 5 cups chicken broth

- 1 cup carrots, diced

- 2 cups cooked chicken, shredded

- ½ cup green spring onions, sliced

- 4 celery ribs, finely chopped

- ½ onion, finely chopped

- 1 tsp garlic powder

- salt and black pepper to taste

- 1 carrot (optional)

*1 cup whole wheat noodle pasta, optional (0.2g in sugar per 100gm, 25g of carbs. Maybe just add 1/2 cup)

Directions:

1. Put all ingredients except the noodles and the cooked chicken in a crock pot, or stove top. Mix them. Cook on low for 6 hours.
2. Add cooked chicken pieces half an hour before serving to heat through thoroughly.
3. Cook noodles and spoon into bowl. Pour soup over the top. Garnish with herbs.

Hungarian Soup

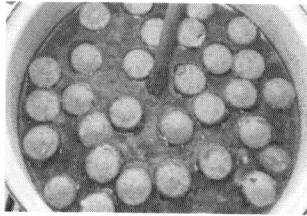

This soup tastes even better the next day!

Ingredients:

- 1/2 large cabbage, sliced

- 3 litres of water or about 13 cups

- 1 small can of tomato puree or tomato paste

- 1 tsp BBQ or Italian style seasoning

- 1 Tbsp salt

- 2 tsp ground black pepper

- 1/2 tsp ground cumin powder

- 1/2 tsp chili flakes, or fresh chili

- 1 red bell pepper

- 2 Tbsp olive oil

- 1 Tbsp low carb flour for thickening

- 2 Tbsp ground paprika

- 1 cup water extra

- 1 cup mashed potato or cauliflower, mashed in the water they were cooked in

- 2 cups smoked sausage of your choice, chopped (salami, cabana, chorizo etc or a blend. Read labels for sugar content)

Directions:

1. Fill a large stock pot with water, sliced cabbage, tomato, seasonings, chili, cumin and bell pepper. Bring to boil, then back to simmer.
2. While that is simmering, fry the flour gently in the oil over a medium heat for about 5 minutes. It should go a golden brown.
3. Turn off heat, stir in the paprika while the pan is still hot and add the extra 1 cup of water. Scrape into stockpot.
4. Stir in mashed cauli or potato and chopped sausage, mixing well.
5. Simmer for about 3/4 hour.
6. Serve in bowls alone or with a crusty whole grain bread.

*Place any leftovers in the fridge as it tastes better the next day.

Pork Fajitas

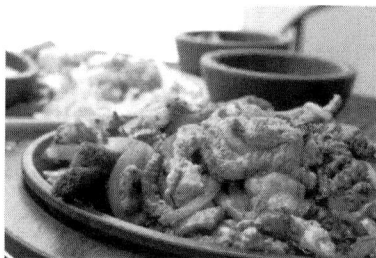

Ingredients:

- 1 lb (450g) pork tenderloin, thinly sliced

- 2 bell peppers, sliced

- 1 onion, sliced

- juice of ½ lime

- 2 Tbsp olive oil

- 1 tsp cayenne pepper

- 1 tsp cumin, ground

- salt and black pepper to taste

Directions:

1. Heat the oil in a large pan over high heat. Add pork, sprinkle salt and black pepper. Cook, stirring for 3 minutes.
2. Add peppers, onion, cayenne and cumin. Cook for 3-5 more minutes. Stir in the lime juice and sauté for 2 more minutes.

http://www.amazon.com/author/peggy-annear

BBQ Chicken Wraps

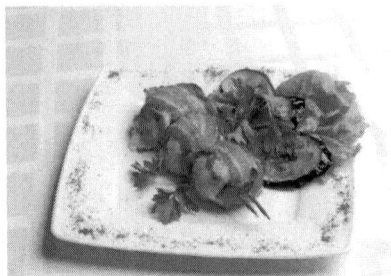

Ingredients

- ½ cup pureed natural apricots, or honey

- ¼ cup apple cider vinegar

- 1 tsp paprika

- 4 skinless chicken thigh or breast fillets

- 8 slices bacon rashers

Directions:

1. Whisk apricot puree or honey, vinegar and smoked paprika together in a saucepan over med-high heat. Simmer for approx. 8 minutes or until thickened.
2. Preheat grill to med-high or use a BBQ.
3. Slice bacon into thirds. Chop chicken into cubes.
4. Placing an individual cube of chicken onto each bacon slice; wrap it around chicken and place onto skewer. Repeat with 3-4 pieces on each skewer.
5. Brush all sides of bacon-wrapped chicken skewers with honey glaze.
6. Cook on hot grill or BBQ turning every 2-3 minutes. Brush with more glaze and cook for about 8-10 minutes.
   *Serve with salad greens & parsley. BBQ eggplant & zucchini or steamed veggies go very nicely too!

Lavender Infused Cutlets

You can soak the cutlets in the marinade first if you wish.

Ingredients:

- 8 lamb cutlets, beef works too

- 1 onion, finely chopped

- 3 Tbsp finely chopped fresh lavender

- 2 Tbsp olive oil

- 1 Tbsp red wine or white vinegar (red wine and white vinegar has nil g of sugar, balsamic 15g, and cider 0.4g of sugar per 100g)

- 1 Tbsp lemon juice

- raw salt and ground black pepper to taste

Directions:

1. Place the cutlets in a large bowl, mix in the onion.
2. Add the lavender.
3. In a small bowl beat together the olive oil, vinegar and lemon juice. Pour over the cutlets. Add the seasonings.
4. Coat the meat.
5. Barbecue the meat, or grill on the stove top basting with the marinade until golden brown, turning as you go.
   Delicious served with a coleslaw, garden salad or just as finger food.

http://www.amazon.com/author/peggy-annear

Mexican Vegetable Fritters

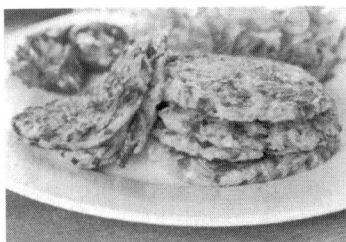

Ingredients:

- 1 cup low carb self raising flour of your choice

- 1/2 can corn, drained, rinsed

- 1 can beans, drained, rinsed

- 2 medium tomatoes, seeds removed, finely chopped

- 1 small bell pepper, finely chopped

- ½ cup milk

- 1 egg, beaten

- 2 Tbsp taco seasoning or BBQ seasoning

- canola oil for frying

- salt and black pepper to taste

Directions:

1. In a bowl mix flour and seasoning. Create a well in the middle.
2. In a small bowl whisk eggs and milk. Pour this mixture in the flour. Whisk until smooth. Add corn, beans, tomatoes and the bell pepper. Mix well.

3. Heat oil in a frying pan over medium heat. Add about ¼ cup of the vegetable mixture to pan. Create a pancake shape with a spatula. Make 4 such fritters on your pan.
4. Cook each of them for 3 minutes, then turn them around and cook for 1 more minute until golden and well done. This recipe should yield around 12 such fritters.
5. Serve hot, with sour cream if desired. Enjoy!

Classic Meatballs

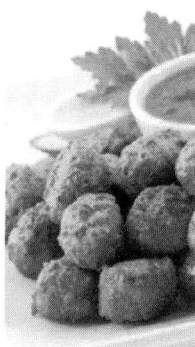

Ingredients: for the meatballs

- 1 pound or about 500gm lean beef mince
- 1 pound or about 500gm lean pork mince
- 1 1/2 Tbsp chopped fresh parsley
- 1 Tbsp chopped fresh oregano or marjoram
- 1 tsp fresh or dried basil
- 2 garlic cloves, crushed and chopped
- 4 small fresh button mushrooms
- 1 egg
- 1 Tbsp olive oil
- black pepper
- raw salt

Ingredients: for the Sauce

- 1 large finely chopped onion
- 150ml dry red wine (about 1g of sugar per 100g)

- 2 cups of canned tomatoes (2.4g of sugar per 100g)
- 1 Tbsp full cream
- 1/2 cup water
- 1 tsp salt
- pinch of ground black pepper
- 1 tsp ground fresh chili (optional)
- 1 tsp fresh or dried oregano
- fresh basil or chives to garnish

Directions: for meatballs

1. Heat the skillet of frying pan to medium and add oil and onion, frying for 2-3 minutes or until slightly golden.
2. Place all the ingredients including the onion into a large bowl and mix thoroughly using your hands. Make sure to "knead" the mixture for a few minutes to bind everything together properly.
3. Wet your hands; roll the meat mixture into small balls the size of a golf ball.
4. Heat the same frying pan to medium high, add some oil and place meatballs into pan. Cook for about 5 -6 minutes on "each side" until done.

Directions: for sauce

1. Heat same pan to medium - add some extra oil to the pan and sauté onion for about 4 minutes (in the same frying pan)
2. De-glaze the pan with the red wine and bring to a simmer. Add the tomatoes, cream, chili, oregano, water, salt and pepper and bring to the simmer again.
3. Serve with cocktail sticks or skewers accompanied with homemade tomato ketchup.

Chili Beef

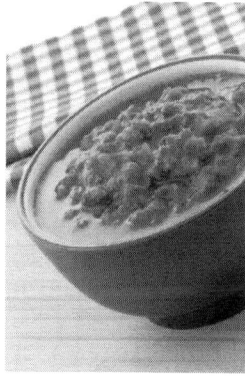

Chili Beef is one of those simple traditional favorites loved by kids and adults! You can add some extra healthy veggies or even vegetable puree for those fussy eaters. Red kidney beans only have 0.3g of sugar, but they have 23g of carbs, so add some if you like.

Ingredients:

- 2 Tbsp olive oil

- 1 diced onion

- 6 stalks of celery (diced)

- 4 garlic cloves (minced)

- 3 1/2 pounds (about 1.3kg) ground beef

- 4 tsp cumin

- 4 tsp chili powder

- 4 tsp oregano

- 2 Tbsp BBQ seasoning

- 2 x 8 oz cans of diced tomatoes

- 1 small can tomato paste or puree

- green chilies to taste

- 4 tsp sea salt

Directions:

1. Using a large pot; fry onions, celery and garlic in oil over med-high heat. Cook for about 4 minutes adding beef and spices and seasonings. Cook for further 5 minutes; stirring constantly.
2. Add tomatoes, paste or puree, chilies and salt. Simmer for about 1 hour.
3. Add a small bunch of chopped parsley at the end of cooking if desired.

*Wonderful as a stand by freezer dinner of lunch!

Beef & Lemongrass Skewers

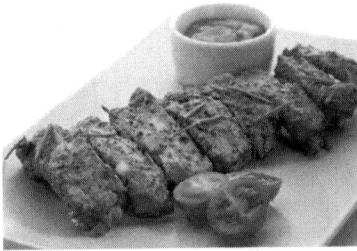

This is very flexible with the meat used and the herbs - I like using rosemary too if it's in the garden. Cilantro/ coriander can be substituted or mixed with rosemary, or even removed all together.

Ingredients:

- 1 pound, about 500 g lean tenderloin beef, cut into small cubes (about 1 1/2 inches)

- 2 cloves garlic, finely chopped

- 4 lemongrass stalks

- 2 Tbsp natural fish sauce (can use anchovies)

- 2 Tbsp sesame oil (nil g of sugar or carbs)

- 2 Tbsp natural maple syrup or Stevia equivalent (maple syrup has 68g of sugar per 100g)

- 1 1/2 tsp ground five spice powder

- 1 small bunch of coriander/cilantro, finely chopped

Directions:

*Soak wooden skewers in water for 1 hour beforehand to stop burning.

1. Prepare the lemongrass by cutting away the top 2 thirds and outer leaves, just using the tender part. Chop finely, or blend.
2. Mix together the garlic, lemongrass, fish sauce, sesame oil, maple syrup, 5 spice and coriander in a bowl.
3. Cut beef into cubes and marinate in the lemongrass mix for at least 20 mins.
4. Thread desired amount onto skewers evenly and fry in oil on stove top or BBQ grill.

*Accompany with favorite dip, salad or salsa. You can either remove or leave on the skewers.

Beef Stoganoff

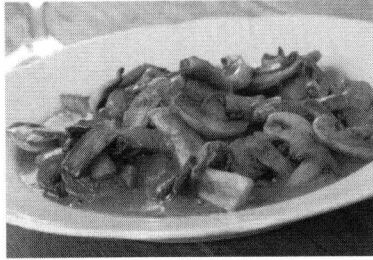

This can be cooked on the stove top or slow cooked in the crockpot. Mushrooms are high in nutrition.

Ingredients:

- 3 pounds or about 1360g, any stewing meat, cubed

- 6 oz or about 170g mushrooms, sliced (about 2g of sugar per 100g and about 4g of carbs)

- 2 cups homemade beef stock (although bought only has around 1.2g of sugar, but not as nutritious)

- ½ cup low carb flour for thickening

- 1 onion, diced

- 1 tsp Tabasco sauce (nil g sugar)

- 1 Tbsp Homemade Tomato Sauce

- 1 tsp salt

- ¼ tsp garlic flakes (fresh will work)

- ¼ tsp black pepper

- ½ cup sour cream, or similar(2.9g of sugar per 100gand 2.9g of carbs)

Directions:

1. Brown the meat and onion in a little oil on the stove top first.
2. Place the meat, onion salt & pepper in a crock pot.
3. In a small bowl combine the beef stock, Tabasco, sauce and garlic. Pour this sauce over the meat. Cook for 8 hours on low or 4 hours on high.
4. Half an hour before serving whisk together the flour and a little of the juice from the crock pot. Pour the sauce back into the crock pot and mix it in briskly. Mix in the mushrooms, and cook on high for 30 minutes.
5. Stir in the cream just before serving.

*Serve with rice or vegetables.

Crockpot Beef Stew

Ingredients:

- 1 Tbsp olive oil

- 1 pound or about 500g lean finely diced or minced beef

- 1 medium brown onion, chopped

- 1 green of red bell pepper, chopped

- 2 cups fresh mixed vegetables such as broccoli, kale, green beans, carrots etc.

- 2 large tins of tomatoes, or about half a dozen fresh home grown.

- 2 cups beef stock and/or water

- Salt, garlic flakes (or fresh) and ground black pepper to taste

Directions:

1. Brown minced beef and onion in frypan. Add bell pepper and cook for a few minutes.
2. Transfer to large heavy saucepan or the crockpot.
3. Add remaining ingredients; cover and cook for 4 hours on low setting or simmer on the stove top for about an hour.

Verde Salsa Beef

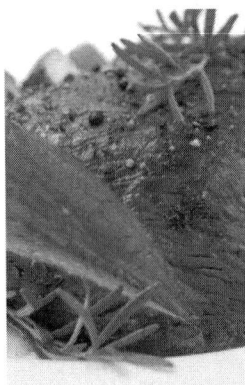

Ingredients:

- 1 sliced tomato (2.6g of sugar per 100g and 3.9g of carbs)
- ½ cup parsley leaves
- ½ cup basil leaves
- 3 cloves garlic
- 2 Tbsp capers (drained)
- 1 anchovy fillet, cut into pieces (nil sugar, nil carbs)
- 1 cup olive oil
- 2 Tbsp fresh lime juice

- salt to taste

- 1 - 2 tsp of black peppercorns (3 color blend is good too)

- 750g (about 25oz) lean sirloin/ fillet steak or similar piece of roasting beef

*Sprinkle with fresh rosemary to garnish

Directions:

1. Purée parsley, basil, garlic, capers, tomato and anchovy fillet in blender; slowly add olive oil until combined. Add lime juice, salt and pepper blending till well combined and smooth. Adjust seasonings to taste and set sauce aside.
2. Season and grill or pan fry steak to your particular preference.
3. When cooked; slice thinly and drizzle with salsa verde. Garnish with some rosemary sprigs or herbs of your choice.

Hungarian Goulash Crockpot

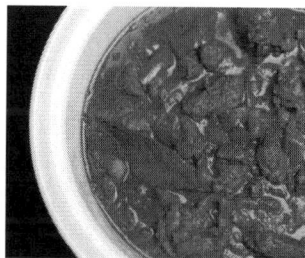

Ingredients:

- 3 1/2 pounds beef, cut into largish cubes

- raw salt and ground black pepper to taste

- 1 Tbsp low carb flour to thicken stew

- 1 Tbsp Hungarian paprika

- 1/4 tsp caraway seeds

- 2 Tbsp coconut oil

- 1 eggplant cut into small pieces or grated (optional. carrot works too)

- 1 large onion, chopped finely

- 3 cloves chopped garlic

- 1 bay leaf

- 1 1/2 red bell peppers cut into chunks

- 1 medium can diced tomatoes

- 1/2 - 1 cup of beef stock if you like more of a soup style (optional)

*A few potatoes can be added to this recipe 3/4 of the way through cooking if desired

Directions:

1. Season the beef with salt, pepper and sprinkle with flour.
2. Heat a large skillet or stock pot to medium high. Brown the meat in half the coconut oil then remove from pan.
3. In same pan add rest of oil and add the onion and garlic, stirring while sautéing for about 3 minutes. Add paprika and caraway seeds for just a minute and stir through, taking care not to burn. This will make the dish bitter.
4. De-glaze the pan with the stock or tomatoes and now add all the remaining ingredients. Cook for about 10 minutes, then transfer to your slow cooker. Usually takes about 6 hours on low. You can add some vegetables like kale or spinach if you wish. If desired this dish can be cooked on the stove top.

Beef and Vegetable Stir Fry

I always use onions or spring onions in this stir fry, although the other veggies are inter changeable.

Ingredients:

- 1 pound or about 16oz of lean beef, pork or chicken, sliced into strips

- 1 Tbsp olive oil for cooking

- 5 cups of assorted bite sized pieces of onion, broccoli, bell capsicum pepper, spring onion, mushrooms, bok choy, carrot. (the vegetables that work are up to you. Use what you have. I change it up with cauliflower, Chinese cabbage, sprouts etc.)

- 2 cloves chopped garlic (optional)

- 3 tsp curry paste (I use Mae Ploy Yellow Curry Paste)

- 1/2 tsp chili (optional - dried flakes or fresh)

- 2 - 3 Tbsp full cream (optional)

- 1 tsp raw salt, or to taste

Directions:

1. Heat wok or frying pan to medium high. Add 1/2 the oil and stir fry the vegetables for about 5 minutes tossing constantly.
2. Add the curry paste, keep stirring for another few minutes till flavors are released. Remove to a dish.
3. Heat wok to high and add remainder oil to the wok and put in the beef strips, garlic and chili. Cook for a further 3 minutes until almost done, then tip all the vegetables back in along with the coconut milk, salt and sesame seeds.

http://www.amazon.com/author/peggy-annear

4. Toss all together for a few minutes more. Serve with fresh herbs, mashed cauliflower or flat bread.

Dijon Pork Chops

Ingredients:

- 4 lean pork chops

- Salt and pepper to taste

- ½ cup Dijon mustard (mustard(s) have about 0.9g of sugar per 100g and about 5g of carbs)

- 1 tsp mustard powder

- 1 tsp dried thyme

- 1 tsp garlic (minced)

- 1 Tbsp olive oil

Directions:

Preheat oven to 425°F (230°C).

1. Season pork chops with salt & pepper.
2. Combine mustard, mustard powder, thyme & garlic in a small bowl. Mix well. Spread evenly over both sides of pork chops.
3. Heat oil in a large frypan over medium-high, add chops and brown for about 2 minutes per side.
4. Transfer chops to baking dish and cook in oven for another 5-8 minutes or until cooked through.
5. Serve over sautéed baby spinach and/or a scrumptious fresh green salad.

Pork & Kale Rolls

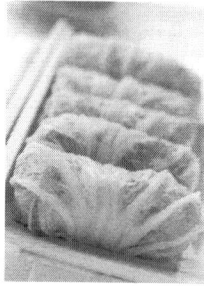

Ingredients:

- 1 pound or about 500g pork tenderloin (any meat leftovers works well)

- 150g kale leaves (cabbage or spinach works well too)

- 2 garlic cloves

- spices for meat: thyme, chili or any other spices you like

- olive oil

Directions:

1. Cut the pork in slices, soften it with a meat mallet. Sprinkle the meat slices generously with a mix of chopped garlic and spices.
2. Blanche the kale leaves, then dry them and put them atop of the pork.
3. Create rolls out of them. Heat up some oil in a frying pan.
4. Once it is hot, fry the rolls on medium to high heat. These can be steamed if desired instead.

Pumpkin Punch

Pumpkin and banana are quite high in sugars, but this recipe has been added for it's nutritional value. Eat in moderation or for a special treat. Another option is to use 1 cup of berries instead of banana. Mix up your own recipes with whatever you have on hand. Get creative, this is how yummy recipes are born!

Ingredients:

- 1/2 cup of pumpkin puree (pumpkin has 2.8g of sugar per 100g and 6g of carbs)

- 1 tsp mixed spice (or cinnamon)

- 1/2 tsp vanilla extract

- 3/4 cup unsweetened almond milk

- 1 chilled or frozen banana or berries (banana is high at 12g of sugar per 100g and 23g carbs)

- 6-7 ice cubes

- honey to taste (I use about 2 tsp)

Directions:

1. Blender until smooth. Garnish with mint and some nutmeg if desired.

Almond Meal Cookies

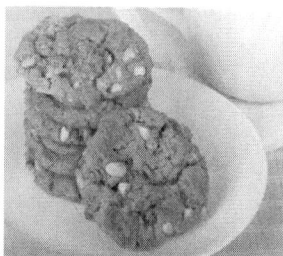

Ingredients:

- 1 Tbsp coconut flour

- 3/4 cup almond meal

- 1 large egg

- 1 Tbsp raw honey, maple syrup or Stevia equivalent

- 1/2 tsp vanilla extract

- 1/3 tsp baking soda

- 4 Tbs coconut or olive oil

- 2 Tbs crushed unsalted cashew nuts (I also use almonds, walnuts or macadamia nuts)

Directions:

Preheat oven to a moderate 350F (180°C).

1. Spray baking tray or sheet with coconut oil spray or line with baking paper.
2. In a medium sized mixer bowl, mix together the almond meal, coconut flour, coconut and baking soda. Add the wet ingredients and mix well.

3. Use a spoon or a small scoop and place smallish "ping pong ball sized" drops of mix onto the tray. With the back of a fork gently press down to flatten.

4. Place in the moderate oven and bake for about 8-10 minutes. **Let the cookies cool for at least 5 minutes** so they can set or firm up.

Each cake - 3.5g Sugar
0.5g Carb

Raspberry Muffins

Ingredients:

- 1 cup almond or low carb flour
- 1 tsp baking powder
- pinch of salt
- 1 cup softened natural butter, or almond butter
- 1 cup fresh raspberries, or blackberries
- ½ cup olive oil
- ¼ cup raw honey, maple syrup or Stevia equivalent
- 3 eggs, whisked
- ¼ cup slivered or flaked almonds

Directions:

Preheat oven to 350°F (180°C).

1. In a medium - large size bowl mix together all dry ingredients: almond flour, baking powder and salt.
2. In another bowl combine butter, honey, oil and eggs mixing well.
3. Gently combine the wet ingredients and raspberries into the dry.
4. Scoop the batter in slightly greased muffin cups (or use paper muffin liners). Cover each muffin with sliced almonds as decoration.
5. Bake for 15-20 minutes.

Fruit Parfait

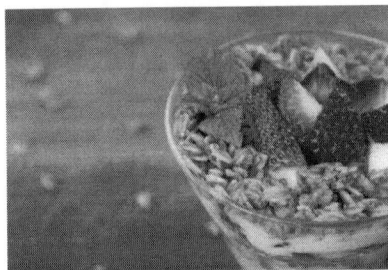

Oats is low in sugar and low in GI making it good for a satisfying breakfast. It is high in carbs but fibre too. So eat in moderation.

Ingredients:

- ¾ cup fruit of your choice (apricot and cranberries are good)

- ½ cup oatmeal (oats has 0.3g of sugar per 100g and 66g of carbs)

- ½ cup skim ricotta

- ½ tsp flavoring (such as almond, vanilla or lemon)

- dash of cinnamon

- dash of nutmeg

Directions:

Preheat the oven to 350°F (180°C).

1. Spread the oats on a baking sheet. Bake for 10 minutes until lightly brown.
2. Mix in cinnamon and nutmeg. Let the oats cool.
3. Meanwhile mix ricotta with your favorite flavoring and cut the fruit in small bite-size pieces.

Once the oats have cooled, alternate layers of oats, ricotta and fruit in a serving bowl. Enjoy!

Roasted Rosemary Almonds

Try any assortment of nuts and seeds you like. Almonds have 4.6g of sugar per 100g and 18g of carbs.

Ingredients:

- 1 1/2 cups raw almonds with skin on (can use other nuts like hazelnuts, cashews and macadamias)

- 1 Tbsp butter

- 1 Tbsp fresh rosemary, minced (use the whole sprig)

- 1 clove of garlic, minced

- salt and ground black pepper to taste

- 2 tsp Worcestershire or Tabasco sauce

Directions:

Preheat oven to 350°F (180°C).

1. In a large non-stick skillet pan heated to medium, fry the rosemary and garlic in the butter or oil for 10 seconds until the aromas are released.
2. Add the almonds and seasoning, stirring quickly for about 1 min, making sure the almonds are coated well with the spice mix. If you want to use seeds, add them last.
3. Pour over the source again mixing quickly for about 1 min. Place the nuts onto a baking tray and bake until the nut are toasted, about 5 to 10 mins.
   *Serve immediately, or cool and place in an airtight container in the refrigerator for up to 2 days.

http://www.amazon.com/author/peggy-annear

Other Good Reads

Low Sugar Smoothies by Peggy Annear

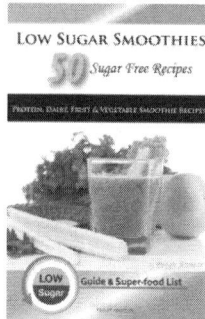

No Sugar Diet by Peggy Annear

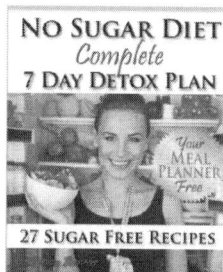

More Low Sugar Recipes, Detox & Diet Plan by Peggy Annear

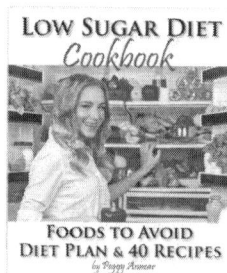

Positive reviews are an author's best friend. If you have enjoyed this book and can spare a minute to **leave a review that would be much appreciated, thank you**.

***

http://www.amazon.com/author/peggy-annear

Notes

Copyright

Sugar Free Recipes: Low Carb Low Sugar Recipes on a Sugar Smart Diet:

Copyright © 2015 by Peggy Annear

Disclaimer: This book is from my experiences gathering nutritional information from USDA and preparing meals including some recipes from friends and variations from other recipes. It has been prepared in good faith, with the goal being to share recipe favorites with others. I am not liable in any way how you choose to use this information as it is an account of my own experiences in the home environment. I have set out to give helpful low sugar recipe ideas. Please consult your doctor or dietician to work out a specific plan for yourself as an individual.

http://www.amazon.com/author/peggy-annear